AF447929

THE NARCISSIST'S PLAYBOOK

The Narcissist's Playbook

Louis Faxan

Copyright © 2024 by Louis Faxan

All rights reserved. No part of this book may be reproduced in any manner whatsoever without written permission except in the case of brief quotations embodied in critical articles and reviews.

First Printing, 2024

Contents

1

Understanding Narcissism

Definition and Characteristics

Narcissism is often misconstrued as mere self-absorption; however, it encompasses a broader spectrum of behaviors and traits that can significantly impact interpersonal dynamics. At its core, narcissism is characterized by an inflated sense of self-importance, a deep need for excessive admiration, and a lack of empathy for others. Narcissists may present themselves as charming and charismatic individuals, which can make it challenging to identify their manipulative tendencies initially. Understanding these defining characteristics is crucial for those dealing with narcissists, as it equips individuals with the insight needed to recognize harmful behaviors before they escalate.

One of the primary traits of a genuine narcissist is their grandiosity, which manifests in numerous ways, including boasting about achievements or exaggerating talents. This self-aggrandizing behavior often leads them to believe they are superior to others, fostering a sense of entitlement. Narcissists may also engage in exploitative behavior, using others to achieve their own goals without regard for the feelings or needs of those they manipulate. In romantic relationships, this can create an uneven dynamic where the narcissist demands constant validation while providing little emotional support in return. Recognizing these traits is essential for individuals who find themselves entangled with narcissistic partners.

In a workplace setting, narcissists can be particularly destructive due to their competitive nature and their tendency to undermine colleagues to elevate their status. They often seek positions of authority, where they can assert control and garner admiration from subordinates and peers alike. Their lack of empathy can lead to toxic work environments, where teamwork and collaboration suffer. Identifying narcissistic behaviors among colleagues or supervisors is vital for maintaining a healthy professional atmosphere and protecting oneself from emotional exploitation.

Narcissism is not limited to overt displays of arrogance; covert narcissism can be equally damaging, albeit more insidious. Covert narcissists tend to present themselves as sensitive or vulnerable, often playing the victim to manipulate others' sympathy. This subtler form of narcissism can be particularly challenging to detect, as it masquerades under the guise of emotional depth and introspection. Understanding the distinction between overt and covert narcissism is essential for recognizing the full spectrum of manipulative behaviors that can occur within friendships and family relationships.

The role of social media in amplifying narcissistic behaviors cannot be overlooked. Platforms that encourage self-promotion and validation can exacerbate the tendencies of narcissists, allowing them to curate and project an idealized version of themselves. This can create an environment where genuine connections are overshadowed by superficial interactions, making it even more difficult for individuals to discern authentic relationships from those characterized by manipulation. By recognizing the defining characteristics of narcissism and understanding its various manifestations, individuals can better navigate their interactions with narcissists in all areas of life, ultimately protecting their mental health and well-being.

The Spectrum of Narcissism

The concept of narcissism exists on a spectrum, ranging from healthy self-esteem to extreme, maladaptive behaviors that can severely impact interpersonal relationships and mental health. At one end of this spectrum, individuals possess a balanced sense of self-worth, which enables them to navigate social situations with confidence and empathy. These individuals can celebrate their achievements without belittling others, fostering positive interactions. However, as one moves along the spectrum toward more pathological traits, the characteristics of narcissism begin to emerge, presenting challenges for those in close proximity to such individuals.

Genuine narcissists often display a combination of overt and covert traits that can be perplexing to those who interact with them. Overt narcissists are typically more recognizable, exhibiting grandiosity, a need for admiration, and a blatant disregard for the feelings of others. In contrast, covert narcissists may present themselves as more sensitive or insecure, yet they still harbor a deep-seated sense of entitlement and can engage in manipulative behaviors. Recognizing these traits is essential for those dealing with narcissists, as the subtlety of covert narcissism can often mask underlying harmful tendencies.

In romantic relationships, identifying narcissistic traits can be particularly challenging due to the emotional investment involved. Narcissists often employ charm and charisma early in a relationship, creating a façade of idealization that can be intoxicating. However, as the relationship progresses, the underlying manipulative behaviors may surface, including gaslighting, emotional unavailability, and a lack of genuine empathy. Understanding the dynamics of narcissism in romantic settings is crucial for individuals seeking to protect their emotional well-being and establish healthier relationships.

The workplace is another arena where narcissism can manifest, influencing group dynamics and overall productivity. Narcissistic individuals may seek power and recognition, often at the expense of colleagues. They might engage in competitive behaviors, undermine others, and create a toxic environment that stifles collaboration. Recognizing these traits early on can help individuals navigate workplace relationships more effectively and foster a healthier organizational culture. Awareness of narcissistic behaviors can empower individuals to set boundaries and advocate for a more supportive work environment.

The rise of social media has further complicated the landscape of narcissism, providing a platform for individuals to showcase their lives in a curated manner that often emphasizes superficial traits. This environment can exacerbate narcissistic behaviors, as individuals may seek validation through likes and followers. For those dealing with narcissists, understanding the impact of social media on behavior is vital, as it can reveal patterns of attention-seeking and self-promotion that may not be as apparent in face-to-face interactions. Recognizing these behaviors can equip individuals with the tools needed to identify and address narcissism in various social contexts, ultimately promoting healthier relationships and mental health.

The Psychology Behind Narcissistic Behavior

Narcissistic behavior is often rooted in a complex interplay of psychological factors that can be traced back to early developmental experiences. Many psychologists suggest that narcissism stems from a combination of innate temperament and environmental influences, particularly during formative years. Children who receive excessive pampering or, conversely, neglect may develop an inflated sense of self-worth as a defense mechanism. This psychological structure serves to shield them from feelings of inadequacy and vulnerability. Understanding these roots can provide clarity for those dealing with narcissists, as it highlights that such behaviors are often not merely an expression of arrogance, but rather a coping strategy for deep-seated insecurities.

Identifying narcissistic traits in romantic relationships requires an understanding of how these behaviors manifest. Narcissists often exhibit a profound need for admiration and validation, frequently demanding attention while simultaneously dismissing their partner's needs. The cycle of idealization and devaluation is common, where the narcissist initially showers their partner with affection before turning critical and manipulative. This push-and-pull dynamic can be bewildering and exhausting for the partner, leading to feelings of confusion and low self-esteem.

Recognizing these patterns is crucial for individuals to regain their sense of self-worth and establish healthier boundaries.

In the workplace, narcissists can create toxic environments that undermine team cohesion and morale. Their self-serving behaviors often manifest as an unwillingness to share credit for successes, a tendency to belittle others, and an insatiable need for recognition. This not only affects colleagues' mental health but can also hinder overall productivity. Understanding the impact of narcissism in professional settings is vital for fostering a collaborative atmosphere. By recognizing these traits in co-workers or supervisors, employees can develop strategies to manage their interactions and protect their own well-being.

The distinction between covert and overt narcissism is essential for accurately identifying narcissistic individuals among friends and family. Overt narcissists are often overtly grandiose and attention-seeking, while covert narcissists may present as shy or introverted, masking their self-centeredness with a facade of vulnerability. Both types, however, share a lack of empathy and a preoccupation with their own needs. Being aware of these different expressions of narcissism can help individuals navigate their relationships more effectively, enabling them to spot manipulative behaviors regardless of the narcissist's outward presentation.

Social media has become a significant arena for revealing narcissistic behavior, as platforms provide an easy outlet for self-promotion and validation. Individuals with narcissistic tendencies often curate their online personas to showcase an idealized version of themselves, seeking affirmation through likes and comments. This behavior can distort perceptions of self-worth, both for the narcissist and their audience. Recognizing the role social media plays in amplifying narcissistic traits offers insight into how these behaviors can infiltrate personal relationships and influence group dynamics. By understanding this connection, individuals can better protect themselves from the negative impact of such behaviors in their social circles.

2

How to Spot Genuine Narcissists

Key Behavioral Indicators

Understanding the key behavioral indicators of narcissism is essential for anyone navigating relationships with narcissistic individuals, whether they are friends, family members, or colleagues. The first significant indicator is an inflated sense of self-importance. Narcissists often exhibit an exaggerated belief in their own superiority, expecting recognition and admiration without commensurate achievements. This trait can be especially pronounced in romantic relationships, where they may demand constant validation and attention from their partners while showing little interest in their partner's needs or feelings.

Another critical behavioral indicator is a pervasive lack of empathy. Narcissists struggle to recognize or care about the emotions of others, which can manifest in dismissive or condescending behavior. In workplace settings, this may translate into a disregard for colleagues' contributions, as they prioritize their own agendas over team dynamics. This lack of empathy often leads to toxic environments where individuals feel undervalued and demoralized, creating challenges in maintaining healthy professional relationships.

Manipulative behavior is another hallmark of narcissism, characterized by deceit and exploitation. Narcissists frequently employ tactics such as gaslighting, where they distort reality to confuse and control their victims. This can occur in various contexts, from family dynamics to friendships, where a narcissist may twist situations to paint themselves as the victim or to shift blame. Recognizing these manipulative patterns is crucial for identifying narcissism, as they can create a cycle of emotional turmoil for those affected.

Social media serves as a revealing platform for narcissistic behavior, amplifying certain traits and tendencies. Individuals with narcissistic inclinations often curate their online presence meticulously, showcasing an idealized version of themselves while seeking validation through likes and comments. This can lead to a distorted perception of self-worth based on external feedback. Understanding how social media influences narcissistic behaviors can help individuals spot red flags in online interactions and relationships.

Lastly, recognizing the impact of narcissism on mental health is vital. The emotional toll of engaging with narcissistic individuals can lead to anxiety, depression, and a diminished sense of self-worth for those on the receiving end of their behavior. By identifying key behavioral indicators, individuals can empower themselves to set boundaries and protect their mental well-being. Knowledge of these traits not only aids in spotting narcissists but also fosters resilience in the face of manipulative behavior.

Common Responses and Reactions

Common responses and reactions to narcissistic behavior often manifest as a range of emotional and psychological effects on those who interact with narcissists. Individuals may experience confusion and self-doubt as they grapple with the unpredictable nature of a narcissist's actions. This emotional turmoil is often compounded by the narcissist's tendency to manipulate conversations, making those around them feel as though their feelings are invalid or exaggerated. The constant alternation between idealization and devaluation can leave friends, family, and colleagues questioning their own perceptions and experiences. This cycle of emotional chaos can lead to a profound sense of instability, as individuals find themselves reacting to the whims of the narcissist rather than responding from a place of personal strength.

In romantic relationships, the reactions to narcissistic behavior can be particularly intense. Partners of narcissists often find themselves caught in a web of emotional highs and lows, where moments of affection and praise are abruptly followed by criticism and neglect. This push-pull dynamic can result in a deep-seated sense of insecurity, as the partner may feel that their worth is dependent on the narcissist's approval. Over time, this can lead to a diminished sense of self and increased anxiety, as individuals become hyper-vigilant to the narcissist's moods and needs, often at the expense of their own well-being. Understanding this pattern is crucial for those seeking to navigate the complexities of narcissistic relationships, as it highlights the importance of setting boundaries and prioritizing self-care.

In the workplace, interactions with narcissists can produce a unique set of reactions among colleagues. The narcissist's need for admiration and control can create a toxic environment, where employees may feel undervalued or manipulated. Common responses include withdrawal from team dynamics, increased stress levels, and a decrease in overall productivity. Those working alongside narcissists might find themselves second-guessing their contributions, as the narcissist often seeks to take credit for the successes of others while deflecting blame for failures. This behavior can lead to a pervasive atmosphere of fear and competition, ultimately undermining team cohesion and morale. Recognizing these reactions is essential for fostering a healthier workplace culture and encouraging open communication.

Friends and family members of narcissists frequently experience a range of emotional responses that can complicate their relationships. Many initially feel sympathy or concern for the narcissist, believing they can help or change them. However, as the manipulative behaviors become more apparent, these individuals may shift to feelings of frustration, anger, or even guilt for not being able to "fix" the situation. This emotional rollercoaster can result in isolation, as friends and family members withdraw from social interactions to protect themselves from further emotional harm. Understanding these common reactions can empower those affected to seek support, whether through therapy or support groups, and to develop strategies that promote healthier interactions with their narcissistic loved ones.

The influence of narcissism extends beyond individual relationships, impacting group dynamics in both personal and professional settings. Common reactions within group contexts often include polarization, where individuals may align with or against the narcissist, creating factions that disrupt cohesion. The narcissist's manipulative tactics may lead to scapegoating, where blame is deflected onto others, further exacerbating tensions within the group. Recognizing these dynamics is crucial for fostering a sense of community and collaboration, as understanding the common responses to narcissistic behavior can help individuals navigate the complexities of their interactions. By cultivating awareness and promoting healthy communication, those dealing with narcissists can work towards creating environments that prioritize mutual respect and emotional safety.

Case Studies of Identified Narcissists

Case studies provide a powerful lens through which to understand the complex behaviors of narcissists, illustrating the varying manifestations of narcissism across different relationships and environments. One such case involves a romantic relationship where one partner exhibited extreme self-centeredness, constantly seeking validation while dismissing the other's needs. The individual would frequently dominate conversations, redirecting discussions back to themselves and their achievements. In moments of conflict, this person would employ gaslighting techniques, making their partner question their own perceptions and feelings, which ultimately led to emotional exhaustion and a gradual loss of self-esteem for the victim.

In the workplace, a manager displayed classic narcissistic traits that affected team dynamics and morale. Colleagues often felt belittled during meetings, as the manager would take credit for their ideas while deflecting any criticism aimed at them. This environment fostered a culture of fear, where employees felt compelled to agree with the manager's decisions regardless of their personal opinions or the well-being of the team. Over time, high turnover rates and decreased productivity became evident, illustrating the detrimental impact of narcissism on professional settings and highlighting the importance of recognizing these traits early.

Among friends and family, another case study reveals the subtlety of covert narcissism. An individual in a social circle appeared amiable and caring on the surface but often engaged in passive-aggressive behavior. They would manipulate situations to elicit sympathy, positioning themselves as the victim in various scenarios. This behavior created an emotional burden on their friends, who felt compelled to support them while struggling with the underlying resentment that grew from the lack of reciprocity. Understanding this dynamic is crucial for those dealing with narcissists, as it showcases how covert narcissists can operate under a guise of normalcy while still causing significant emotional harm.

The role of social media in revealing narcissistic behavior has become increasingly significant in modern interactions. One case involved an individual who meticulously curated their online presence, constantly sharing posts that highlighted their successes and glamorous lifestyle. This individual's need for validation through likes and comments became apparent, often leading to distress when engagement fell short of expectations. Friends noticed a pattern of self-promotion that overshadowed genuine connections, raising concerns about the authenticity of their relationships. This case underscores the importance of examining social media behavior as a potential indicator of narcissistic traits.

Lastly, the impact of narcissism on mental health is evident in a case where a person struggled to maintain relationships due to their overt narcissistic tendencies. Their interactions were characterized by a lack of empathy, leading to friends and family distancing themselves over time. The narcissist often displayed a façade of confidence, masking deep-seated insecurities and a fear of abandonment. This emotional turmoil not only affected those around them but also led to a cycle of anxiety and depression within the narcissist themselves. Recognizing these behaviors and their repercussions can empower individuals to navigate their interactions more effectively and prioritize their mental health in the process.

3

Narcissistic Traits in Romantic Relationships

Signs of Narcissism in Partners

Identifying narcissistic traits in romantic relationships can be crucial for safeguarding one's emotional well-being. A common sign of narcissism in partners is an excessive need for admiration and validation. This behavior often manifests as constant fishing for compliments or displaying an inflated sense of self-importance. Partners may frequently talk about their achievements, expecting recognition and praise without reciprocating genuine interest in their partner's life. This one-sided dynamic can create an imbalance in the relationship, leaving the non-narcissistic partner feeling undervalued and emotionally drained.

Another hallmark of narcissism is a lack of empathy. Narcissistic partners often struggle to understand or care about their partner's feelings or needs. They may dismiss concerns or emotions as trivial, leading to a pattern of emotional neglect. When conflicts arise, a narcissistic partner might prioritize their own perspective, exhibiting an unwillingness to engage in constructive dialogue or compromise. This behavior can leave the other partner feeling isolated, as their experiences and emotions are continuously sidelined.

Manipulative behavior is also prevalent among narcissistic partners. They may use tactics such as gaslighting, where they distort reality to make their partner question their perceptions or memories. This manipulation can create confusion and self-doubt, making it difficult for the non-narcissistic partner to maintain a clear sense of self. Additionally, narcissistic partners may employ guilt-tripping or blame-shifting to evade responsibility for their actions, further entrenching their partner in a cycle of self-blame and anxiety.

Social media usage can be another indicator of narcissistic behavior in partners. Excessive posting about their life, achievements, or possessions, often with an emphasis on garnering likes and attention, can signal a deep-seated need for external validation. They may curate their online persona meticulously, using it as a tool to project an idealized image that may not reflect reality. This behavior not only reflects a narcissistic trait but can also create a competitive atmosphere within the relationship, as the non-narcissistic partner may feel pressured to keep up with this façade.

Finally, the impact of a narcissistic partner on mental health cannot be overstated. The emotional toll of consistently navigating a relationship marked by manipulation, lack of empathy, and self-centeredness can lead to anxiety, depression, and diminished self-esteem. Recognizing these signs is essential for those dealing with narcissists, as awareness can empower individuals to make informed decisions about their relationships. Establishing boundaries and seeking support can be vital steps in reclaiming one's emotional landscape and fostering healthier connections.

Red Flags During Courtship

Red flags during courtship often serve as critical indicators of potential narcissistic tendencies, especially in romantic relationships. One of the most telling signs is an overwhelming focus on self. A partner who constantly redirects conversations to their achievements or experiences may display traits of narcissism. This self-centeredness not only stifles genuine connection but can also create an environment where your feelings and thoughts are undervalued. Pay attention to how often your partner listens to you versus how frequently they share their own stories; a significant imbalance may suggest a lack of empathy, a core characteristic of narcissistic personalities.

Another warning sign during courtship is the tendency to idealize and devalue partners rapidly. Initially, a narcissist may shower their partner with affection, compliments, and attention, which can feel intoxicating. However, this phase often transitions abruptly to criticism and contempt. This pattern of idealization followed by devaluation can lead to emotional whiplash and confusion, making it difficult for the partner to maintain a stable sense of self-worth. Recognizing this cycle early on can help you avoid deeper emotional entanglements that might leave you feeling insecure and unworthy.

Control and manipulation are also significant red flags in a budding relationship. A narcissistic partner may exhibit behaviors such as isolating you from friends and family or attempting to dictate your choices, whether they relate to personal interests or social engagements. This controlling behavior often masquerades as concern or love but serves to establish dominance. Being aware of how your partner reacts when you express independence or assert your own opinions is crucial. If their response is defensive or dismissive, it may indicate a deeper issue rooted in narcissistic tendencies.

Additionally, the use of social media can unveil narcissistic traits during courtship. If your partner frequently posts about their achievements, appearance, or lifestyle while engaging in excessive self-promotion, this may point to a need for validation that is characteristic of narcissism. Monitoring how they interact with others online—whether they respond to criticism defensively or engage in attention-seeking behavior—can provide insight into their personality. Such behaviors can have long-lasting implications, particularly if they reflect a pattern of seeking external validation rather than fostering intimate connections.

Finally, understanding the impact of narcissism on mental health is paramount. Many individuals who become involved with narcissists may experience increased anxiety, depression, and feelings of inadequacy. The emotional toll of navigating a relationship marked by manipulative behaviors can be profound, often leading to a diminished sense of self-worth. Recognizing these red flags early in courtship can empower individuals to make informed decisions about their relationships and prioritize their emotional well-being. By maintaining awareness of these warning signs, you can protect yourself from the potential pitfalls of a relationship with a narcissist.

Long-term Impacts on Relationships

The long-term impacts of relationships characterized by narcissistic behavior are profound and multifaceted, affecting not only individual mental health but also the dynamics within families, friendships, and workplaces. Individuals entangled with narcissists often experience a gradual erosion of their self-esteem and sense of identity. This depletion is frequently a result of persistent gaslighting, manipulation, and emotional abuse, which can leave victims questioning their perceptions and worth. Over time, the constant need to accommodate the narcissist's demands and fluctuations in mood can lead to chronic stress and anxiety, undermining overall mental well-being.

In romantic relationships, the consequences of narcissism can be particularly damaging. Partners of narcissists often find themselves trapped in a cycle of idealization and devaluation, which can create an unstable emotional environment. Initially, they may experience intense affection and admiration, only to be met with criticism and neglect as the relationship progresses. This unpredictability can foster a deep-seated fear of abandonment, prompting victims to cling to the relationship despite its toxicity. Such dynamics not only hinder personal growth but also instill a lasting fear of intimacy and vulnerability in future relationships.

Narcissism also significantly impacts friendships and familial bonds. When a narcissist is part of a family unit or social circle, their need for admiration and control can create rifts and foster resentment among other members. Genuine relationships often suffer as the narcissist monopolizes attention and emotional resources, leaving others feeling undervalued and unheard. Over time, this can lead to a breakdown of trust and communication, as those around the narcissist may feel compelled to mask their true feelings to avoid conflict or further manipulation. The burden of such dynamics often results in estrangement or superficial relationships that lack depth and authenticity.

In professional settings, the presence of narcissistic individuals can disrupt teamwork and morale. Narcissists often prioritize their own success over collective goals, leading to a toxic work environment where collaboration is stifled. Their tendency to undermine colleagues and take credit for others' work can create an atmosphere of distrust and competition. This not only affects individual job satisfaction but can also impact overall productivity, as team members become demotivated and disengaged. The long-term effects of such an environment can include high turnover rates and a culture of fear, which stifles innovation and growth.

Lastly, the role of social media in exposing narcissistic behaviors cannot be overlooked. Online platforms often amplify narcissistic tendencies by providing a stage for self-promotion and validation. The constant pursuit of likes and followers can exacerbate the existing issues within relationships, as individuals may feel compelled to present a curated version of their lives that aligns with narcissistic ideals. This can lead to further isolation and disconnection from genuine relationships, as the line between authenticity and performance blurs. Ultimately, the long-term impacts of narcissistic relationships are far-reaching, affecting not only the individuals directly involved but also their social networks and communities.

4

Recognizing Narcissism in the Workplace

Identifying Narcissistic Colleagues

Identifying narcissistic colleagues requires a keen understanding of specific behavioral traits that distinguish them from others in the work-place. Narcissists often present themselves as charismatic and self-assured, which can initially make them seem appealing. However, their underlying motives typically revolve around self-interest, manipulation, and a lack of genuine empathy for others. Observing patterns in how these individuals interact with colleagues can provide critical insights into their narcissistic tendencies. Look for signs of excessive self-promotion, a tendency to dominate conversations, and a dismissive attitude toward the input and achievements of others.

One key characteristic of narcissistic colleagues is their need for admiration and validation. They often seek out praise and recognition, sometimes to the detriment of team cohesion. This can manifest in various ways, such as taking credit for group successes or frequently steering discussions back to their accomplishments. Furthermore, they may engage in gaslighting, where they distort facts and manipulate situations to maintain their self-image. Recognizing these behaviors early on can help you navigate the complexities of working alongside a narcissist, allowing you to set appropriate boundaries and protect your own mental well-being.

Narcissists are also adept at creating an illusion of superiority, which can be particularly evident in competitive work environments. They may engage in belittling others or undermining colleagues to elevate their own status. This can lead to a toxic atmosphere where collaboration is stifled, and morale plummets. Pay attention to how colleagues react to this individual; a pattern of fear, resentment, or discomfort can indicate the presence of a narcissistic personality. Being aware of the dynamic can empower you to address issues diplomatically and foster a healthier work environment.

Understanding the difference between overt and covert narcissism is crucial in identifying narcissistic colleagues. Overt narcissists are typically more obvious in their grandiosity and entitlement, making their behaviors easier to spot. In contrast, covert narcissists may present as shy or introverted while still exhibiting manipulative behaviors, such as passive-aggressiveness or playing the victim. This distinction is vital to recognize, as it can affect how colleagues respond to and engage with these individuals. Being able to identify both forms allows for a more nuanced understanding of workplace dynamics influenced by narcissism.

Finally, the role of social media cannot be underestimated when identifying narcissistic traits in colleagues. Many narcissists curate their online presence to project an image of success and admiration, often seeking validation through likes and comments. This behavior can extend into the workplace, where they may leverage social media to further their agendas or manipulate perceptions. Monitoring how colleagues interact with social media can provide additional context for their narcissistic tendencies, offering insights into their need for external validation. By combining these observations of behavior, communication, and social media presence, you can more effectively identify narcissistic colleagues and mitigate their impact on your professional life.

Workplace Manipulation Tactics

Workplace manipulation tactics employed by narcissists can create a toxic environment that undermines productivity and morale. These individuals often use insidious strategies to maintain control and assert dominance over their colleagues. Common tactics include gaslighting, where the narcissist distorts reality to make others doubt their perceptions, and triangulation, which involves creating conflict between coworkers to isolate the target and consolidate power. Recognizing these behaviors is crucial for anyone navigating a workplace affected by narcissistic dynamics.

Another prevalent tactic is the use of charm and flattery. Narcissists often project a charismatic persona, initially winning over colleagues with compliments and seemingly genuine interest. However, this charm is typically superficial and serves to manipulate others into a position of dependence. Once trust is established, they may exploit this relationship for personal gain, often leaving their victims feeling confused and disillusioned. Understanding this cycle of manipulation can help individuals maintain a critical perspective on their interactions.

Narcissists may also engage in passive-aggressive behaviors, which can be particularly damaging in a professional setting. Instead of confronting issues directly, they may express hostility through indirect means, such as withholding information, sabotaging projects, or giving backhanded compliments. This can create an atmosphere of fear and uncertainty, where team members feel they must tread carefully to avoid provoking the narcissist's ire. Identifying these tactics is essential for fostering a healthier workplace culture.

Moreover, narcissists often play the victim, shifting blame onto others to evade responsibility for their actions. This tactic allows them to manipulate colleagues into feeling guilty or sympathetic, diverting attention from their own shortcomings. By portraying themselves as misunderstood or unfairly treated, they can garner support and create alliances that further entrench their position within the workplace hierarchy.

Awareness of this behavior can empower colleagues to challenge these narratives and hold narcissists accountable for their actions.

Finally, it is important to recognize the long-term impact of narcissistic manipulation on mental health and overall team dynamics. Victims of workplace narcissism may experience increased stress, anxiety, and a decline in self-esteem. This not only affects individual well-being but can also lead to decreased collaboration and innovation within teams. By equipping oneself with the knowledge to identify workplace manipulation tactics, individuals can better protect their mental health and advocate for a more supportive and respectful work environment.

Navigating the Challenges of a Narcissistic Boss

Navigating the challenges posed by a narcissistic boss can be a daunting task that significantly impacts both professional development and workplace morale. Narcissistic leaders often exhibit traits such as a relentless need for admiration, a lack of empathy, and a tendency to manipulate others for their gain. These behaviors can create a toxic work environment where employees feel undervalued and exploited. Understanding these dynamics is crucial in formulating effective strategies to cope with and counteract the negative effects of such leadership.

One of the first steps in managing a relationship with a narcissistic boss is to develop a keen awareness of their patterns of behavior. Recognizing traits such as an excessive focus on their own achievements, a dismissive attitude toward employees' contributions, and an inclination to take credit for others' work can help clarify the nature of their narcissism. Additionally, observing how they react to criticism or failure can provide insights into their fragile self-esteem and the subsequent defensive behaviors they may exhibit. This awareness not only aids in anticipating potential conflicts but also informs how to communicate effectively with them.

Communicating with a narcissistic boss requires a strategic approach. It is essential to frame feedback and suggestions in a way that appeals to their ego. This may involve highlighting how certain ideas or initiatives can enhance their reputation or contribute to the organization's success, thereby aligning your objectives with their need for validation. Furthermore, maintaining professionalism and avoiding direct confrontations can minimize the likelihood of triggering their defensiveness. By carefully managing interactions, employees can navigate the complexities of the relationship while maintaining their own dignity and well-being.

Setting boundaries is another critical aspect of dealing with a narcissistic boss. Establishing clear limits around work expectations and personal interactions helps protect one's mental health from the potential onslaught of manipulation and emotional exploitation. It is vital to recognize the importance of self-care and to seek support from colleagues or mentors who understand the challenges posed by narcissism. Creating a network of trusted individuals can provide emotional resilience and practical advice on how to handle difficult situations effectively.

Finally, when the situation becomes intolerable, considering the long-term implications of remaining in such an environment is essential. If the narcissistic behavior leads to a toxic atmosphere that adversely affects your mental health, it may be necessary to explore other job opportunities or seek a transfer within the organization. Remembering that your professional worth is not defined by a narcissistic boss's perception is crucial. Prioritizing your mental health and career growth can empower you to make decisions that align with your values and aspirations, ultimately leading to a more fulfilling professional life.

5

Spotting Narcissists Among Friends and Family

Behavioral Patterns in Close Relationships

Behavioral patterns in close relationships often reveal the underlying dynamics that can signal the presence of narcissism. Individuals in close relationships with narcissists frequently experience a cycle of idealization, devaluation, and discard. In the initial stages, the narcissist may shower their partner with attention and affection, creating a sense of euphoria. This idealization phase can be intoxicating, making it difficult for the partner to recognize any red flags. However, as the relationship progresses, the narcissist's need for control and validation often leads to a gradual shift toward devaluation. Partners may find themselves criticized, belittled, or manipulated, creating a confusing and emotionally tumultuous environment.

In romantic relationships, identifying narcissistic traits can be particularly challenging due to the emotional investment often involved. Narcissists may employ charm and charisma to mask their true intentions, leaving their partners feeling unworthy and dependent. This dependency is a key tactic used by narcissists to maintain power within the relationship. Victims may begin to doubt their own perceptions and feelings, as the narcissist skillfully twists reality to serve their narrative. Recognizing these patterns can empower individuals to reclaim their sense of self and establish healthier boundaries.

The workplace presents another arena in which narcissistic behavior can manifest, often impacting team dynamics and overall morale. Narcissistic colleagues or superiors may exhibit a lack of empathy, taking credit for others' work while avoiding accountability for their own shortcomings. This can create a toxic environment where collaboration is stifled, and individuals feel undervalued. Understanding the signs of narcissism in professional settings is crucial for fostering a healthier workplace culture. Employees should be encouraged to document interactions and seek support when faced with manipulative behaviors, thus reducing the narcissist's influence.

Among friends and family, spotting narcissism can be equally complex. The emotional ties that bind individuals to narcissistic family members or friends can obscure the reality of their behavior. Narcissists often manipulate those closest to them through guilt, obligation, or emotional blackmail, making it difficult for victims to break free from these relationships. Family gatherings or social events may become battlegrounds for attention and validation, leaving others feeling emotionally drained and unsupported. Recognizing these patterns can help individuals create distance and protect their own mental wellbeing.

The role of social media in revealing narcissistic behavior cannot be overlooked. Platforms that encourage self-promotion and validation can amplify narcissistic tendencies, allowing individuals to curate their image while disregarding authentic connections. The constant need for likes, comments, and attention can exacerbate existing narcissistic traits, making it essential for individuals to remain vigilant. By analyzing online interactions and recognizing the signs of narcissistic behavior, individuals can better navigate their relationships both online and offline, ultimately fostering healthier connections.

Emotional Manipulation Tactics

Emotional manipulation is a core tactic employed by narcissists to maintain control and power over their victims. By exploiting the emotions of others, narcissists can create a dynamic where they are seen as the victim or the hero, depending on what serves their interests. Understanding these tactics is crucial for those dealing with narcissists, as it allows individuals to recognize when they are being manipulated and to respond effectively. Emotional manipulation often includes gaslighting, guilt-tripping, and love bombing, each designed to destabilize the target's sense of reality and self-worth.

Gaslighting is one of the most insidious forms of emotional manipulation. It involves the narcissist denying reality, causing the victim to doubt their perceptions and memories. This tactic effectively shifts the blame onto the victim, making them feel confused and insecure. In romantic relationships, for instance, a partner may dismiss concerns about their behavior, insisting the victim is overreacting or misremembering events. This erosion of trust in one's own thoughts can lead to significant psychological distress and can be particularly damaging in intimate relationships where trust and communication are paramount.

Guilt-tripping is another common tactic used by narcissists to manipulate others emotionally. By invoking feelings of guilt, narcissists can compel their victims to conform to their demands or expectations. For example, a narcissistic friend may remind you of how much they have done for you, implying that any refusal to comply with their wishes is a betrayal. This tactic not only enforces compliance but also fosters a sense of obligation that can be difficult to navigate. In familial settings, this can manifest as emotional blackmail, where the narcissist leverages family loyalty to control behaviors and decisions.

Love bombing, characterized by an overwhelming display of affection and attention, is often used as a means to draw victims into a narcissistic orbit. Initially, this behavior may feel flattering and intoxicating, leading individuals to believe they have found a deeply caring partner or friend. However, as the relationship progresses, the intensity of this affection typically diminishes, and the narcissist may withdraw their attention, leaving the victim feeling confused and desperate for validation. This cycle reinforces the narcissist's control, as the victim learns to associate their self-worth with the narcissist's approval.

Recognizing these emotional manipulation tactics is essential for anyone navigating relationships with narcissists. By understanding how these behaviors manifest, individuals can develop strategies to protect themselves and their mental health. Setting clear boundaries, seeking support from trusted friends or professionals, and remaining grounded in one's own reality can help mitigate the impact of emotional manipulation. Ultimately, awareness of these tactics empowers individuals to reclaim their autonomy and foster healthier, more balanced relationships.

Strategies for Managing Narcissistic Family Dynamics

Effective management of narcissistic family dynamics requires a strategic approach that recognizes the unique challenges posed by such relationships. One of the most critical strategies is maintaining clear boundaries. Establishing and enforcing personal limits helps protect one's emotional well-being and prevents narcissistic individuals from overstepping. It is essential to communicate these boundaries assertively and consistently, as narcissists often test limits to gauge how much control they can exert. By standing firm, family members can minimize the emotional turmoil that often accompanies interactions with a narcissistic relative.

Another vital strategy is to practice emotional detachment. While this may seem emotionally challenging, it is necessary to reduce the impact of the narcissist's behavior on one's mental health. This involves recognizing that the narcissistic individual's actions and words stem from their psychological issues rather than a reflection of one's worth. By reframing interactions and viewing them through this lens, family members can cultivate a sense of distance that fosters resilience. This emotional detachment does not imply a lack of care, but rather a protective measure that allows individuals to engage without becoming overly affected by the narcissist's manipulations.

Communication plays a pivotal role in managing these dynamics. Using non-confrontational language when addressing issues can help to avoid triggering defensive reactions from the narcissist. It is advisable to focus on "I" statements rather than "you" statements, which can lead to blame and escalation. For instance, saying "I feel overwhelmed when decisions are made without my input" is more constructive than "You never listen to me." This approach fosters a more collaborative atmosphere, potentially leading to more productive discussions, even with challenging individuals.

In addition to these strategies, seeking support from outside sources can provide essential relief and perspective. Connecting with others who understand the complexities of narcissistic relationships, whether through support groups or therapy, can offer valuable insights and coping mechanisms. These external resources can help family members process their experiences, validate their feelings, and reinforce their strategies for dealing with narcissists. This support network can serve as a buffer against the isolation and confusion that often accompany interactions with narcissistic family members.

Finally, it is important to recognize when professional intervention is necessary. If the dynamics become overwhelmingly toxic or harmful, seeking guidance from a mental health professional can be crucial. A therapist can help individuals develop tailored strategies for managing interactions with narcissists and provide a safe space to explore the emotional ramifications of these relationships. Understanding the nuances of narcissistic behavior and its impact on family dynamics can empower individuals to navigate these challenges with greater confidence and clarity.

6

Understanding Covert vs. Overt Narcissism

Characteristics of Overt Narcissism

Overt narcissism is characterized by a clear and pronounced display of self-importance and entitlement. Individuals exhibiting overt narcissism often seek to be the center of attention, drawing energy and validation from others through grandiose behaviors and statements. They may boast about their achievements, exaggerate their talents, and demand recognition and admiration from those around them. This outward display can manifest in various settings, whether in social gatherings, romantic relationships, or professional environments, making it crucial for those dealing with narcissists to recognize these traits early on.

In romantic relationships, overt narcissists often engage in behaviors that prioritize their needs and desires above all else. They may charm their partners initially with charisma and confidence, but over time, their self-centeredness becomes apparent. Communication often revolves around them, with little interest in their partner's feelings or accomplishments. This imbalance can lead to emotional distress for the partner, who may feel invisible or unappreciated. Identifying these traits early in a relationship is vital to avoid becoming ensnared in a cycle of emotional manipulation.

In the workplace, overt narcissists can be particularly challenging to navigate. They may seek leadership positions and often thrive in environments that reward assertiveness and self-promotion. Colleagues may find themselves competing for recognition, as overt narcissists frequently undermine others to elevate their status. Their behavior can create a toxic work atmosphere, leading to high turnover rates and decreased morale among team members. Recognizing these patterns is essential for maintaining a healthy work environment and ensuring that boundaries are established to protect against manipulative tactics.

Among friends and family, overt narcissism can lead to strained relationships and feelings of resentment. These individuals often demand loyalty and admiration, expecting others to cater to their needs without reciprocation. This dynamic can leave friends and family members feeling drained and unvalued, as their own experiences and emotions are overshadowed by the narcissist's need for attention. Awareness of these characteristics can help individuals set boundaries and engage in healthier interactions, ultimately safeguarding their emotional well-being.

Social media serves as a powerful amplifier of overt narcissistic behavior, allowing individuals to curate their image and seek validation in real-time. Overt narcissists often use platforms to showcase their lives in an exaggerated manner, highlighting perceived successes while downplaying any failures. This constant need for approval can lead to a distorted sense of self-worth and foster a culture of comparison among peers. Understanding the role of social media in revealing these traits can aid in identifying overt narcissism, enabling individuals to navigate their relationships with greater awareness and discernment.

Characteristics of Covert Narcissism

Covert narcissism, often overshadowed by its more overt counterpart, manifests through subtle and insidious behaviors that can be challenging to identify. Unlike overt narcissists, who openly seek admiration and validation, covert narcissists often present themselves as shy, sensitive, or self-effacing, masking their need for attention beneath a façade of humility. This deceptive exterior allows them to elicit sympathy and support from those around them while simultaneously manipulating interpersonal dynamics to maintain control. Recognizing these characteristics is essential for those seeking to understand and navigate relationships with covert narcissists.

One of the defining traits of covert narcissism is a profound sense of victimhood. Covert narcissists frequently portray themselves as misunderstood or persecuted, leading others to feel pity or a sense of obligation to help them. This victim mentality serves as a powerful tool, enabling them to manipulate their environment and elicit emotional responses from friends, family, and colleagues. By positioning themselves as the victim, they deflect attention from their own shortcomings and redirect focus onto the perceived injustices they face, thereby maintaining a control that is both subtle and effective.

In romantic relationships, covert narcissists often engage in behaviors that are emotionally manipulative, such as gaslighting or passive-aggressive tactics. They may downplay their partners' feelings or achievements, creating an environment where the partner feels inadequate or overly dependent on the narcissist for validation. This dynamic can lead to significant emotional distress for the partner, as they struggle to navigate the covert narcissist's shifting moods and expectations. Understanding this aspect of covert narcissism is crucial for individuals who find themselves entangled in such relationships, allowing them to recognize unhealthy patterns and seek healthier interactions.

In workplace settings, covert narcissism can manifest through a blend of charm and undermining behavior. These individuals may present themselves as supportive colleagues while simultaneously engaging in backhanded compliments or sabotaging others' work. This duality can create a toxic work environment where competition and mistrust flourish. Recognizing covert narcissistic traits in professional relationships can empower individuals to establish boundaries and protect their mental well-being, fostering a more positive workplace culture where collaboration is prioritized over manipulation.

Covert narcissists also leverage social media to curate their image, often portraying a life filled with accomplishments and emotional depth while masking their underlying insecurities. The carefully crafted online personas can obscure their true nature and further complicate the process of identifying narcissistic traits. For those navigating friendships or familial relationships with covert narcissists, understanding the discrepancies between online portrayals and real-life behavior is essential. This awareness can guide individuals in discerning genuine connections from those that are more superficial and manipulative, ultimately aiding in establishing healthier relationships and fostering personal growth.

Impact on Relationships and Interactions

The presence of narcissistic individuals in one's life can significantly alter the dynamics of relationships and interactions. Whether in a romantic partnership, friendship, or workplace environment, the traits of narcissism often manifest through manipulation, lack of empathy, and a constant need for validation. These behaviors can create an imbalance in relationships, leading to confusion and emotional distress for those on the receiving end. Understanding how these traits affect interpersonal connections can empower individuals to recognize and respond to damaging behaviors effectively.

In romantic relationships, narcissists often charm their partners with an initial display of affection and attention, creating an illusion of intimacy. However, as the relationship progresses, the narcissistic traits become more pronounced, characterized by emotional unavailability, gaslighting, and emotional withdrawal. Partners may find themselves constantly questioning their worth and feeling responsible for the narcissist's emotional state. This dynamic can result in a cycle of dependency and manipulation, where one partner's needs are consistently overlooked, leading to long-term dissatisfaction and erosion of self-esteem.

Among friends and family, narcissism can introduce a toxic element that alters the fundamental nature of these relationships. Narcissists may demand excessive attention and validation from loved ones, often at the expense of others' feelings and needs. This behavior can alienate friends and family members, who may feel undervalued or exploited. Recognizing these patterns is crucial in maintaining healthy boundaries. Those dealing with narcissists must learn to assert their needs while understanding that the narcissist's behavior is more about their insecurities than a reflection of the individuals around them.

In professional settings, narcissism can undermine team dynamics and create a hostile work environment. Narcissistic colleagues or superiors may engage in self-promotion at the expense of team cohesion, often taking credit for others' work while deflecting blame for failures. This behavior fosters an atmosphere of distrust and competition, ultimately hampering productivity and morale. Developing strategies to address and manage interactions with narcissistic individuals in the workplace is essential for maintaining a functional and supportive work environment.

The rise of social media has further complicated the landscape of relationships affected by narcissism. Platforms that encourage self-promotion can amplify narcissistic tendencies, as individuals curate their online personas to seek validation. This constant comparison can lead to feelings of inadequacy and anxiety among those who interact with narcissists online. Understanding the role of social media in revealing narcissistic behavior is vital for individuals navigating these interactions, as it provides context for the behaviors they observe. By recognizing these patterns, individuals can better protect their mental health and engage with others in a more informed and resilient manner.

The Role of Social Media in Revealing Narcissistic

Social Media Profiles as Indicators

Social media profiles serve as a revealing window into the personality traits and behaviors of individuals, particularly when it comes to identifying narcissistic tendencies. For those dealing with narcissists, understanding how to read these profiles can be crucial for navigating relationships effectively. Narcissists often curate their online presence meticulously, showcasing an idealized version of themselves. This curated image typically emphasizes superficial aspects such as physical appearance, accomplishments, and social status, while downplaying any vulnerability or authenticity. By closely examining the content shared on social media, one can often identify patterns indicative of narcissistic behavior.

One of the most prominent indicators of narcissism on social media is the frequency and nature of self-promotion. Narcissists tend to post an excessive amount of photos and updates that highlight their achievements, beauty, or lifestyle. They often seek validation through likes and comments, revealing an underlying need for external affirmation. This behavior can manifest in the form of constant bragging about personal successes, luxurious vacations, or social events, all designed to project an image of superiority. Individuals dealing with such personalities should recognize that this behavior is not merely a reflection of confidence, but often a deep-seated insecurity that drives the need for admiration.

In romantic relationships, social media interactions can further reveal narcissistic traits. A partner's profile might display a pattern of possessiveness or jealousy, particularly if they frequently monitor or comment on their partner's posts. Narcissists may also use social media as a tool for manipulation, creating narratives that paint themselves in a positive light while disparaging others, including their partners. This can lead to a distorted perception of the relationship, where the narcissist appears charming or desirable to outsiders, while the reality may involve emotional manipulation and a lack of genuine connection.

In workplace settings, social media profiles can also provide insights into an individual's narcissistic traits. Colleagues who frequently engage in self-aggrandizing behavior or who exhibit a blatant disregard for others' contributions may display classic signs of narcissism. The way they present themselves online, often highlighting their achievements while minimizing teamwork or collaboration, can be a red flag. Additionally, their interactions with others on these platforms may reveal a tendency to belittle peers or undermine their accomplishments, further illustrating the impact of narcissism on professional dynamics.

Lastly, social media can serve as a platform for both overt and covert narcissism. Overt narcissists are usually straightforward in their self-promotion and attention-seeking behaviors, while covert narcissists may employ subtler tactics, such as passive-aggressive posts or indirect pleas for sympathy. Recognizing these differing styles can help individuals identify manipulative behaviors more effectively. By remaining vigilant and discerning in the face of social media portrayals, those dealing with narcissists can gain valuable insights into the underlying dynamics of their relationships, empowering them to respond appropriately and protect their mental health.

Online Behavior and Narcissistic Traits

Online behavior is a powerful lens through which we can examine narcissistic traits, as digital interactions often amplify certain characteristics inherent in narcissism. The virtual world provides a platform for individuals to curate their identities and present an idealized version of themselves, making it especially relevant for those dealing with narcissists. Online interactions can reveal patterns of behavior that may not be as visible in face-to-face relationships. For instance, individuals with narcissistic tendencies often engage in self-promotional activities, posting content that highlights their achievements, appearance, or lifestyle while neglecting to engage meaningfully with others.

Social media serves as a breeding ground for narcissistic traits, where validation through likes, comments, and shares can reinforce a person's self-centered behaviors. Narcissists may use these platforms to seek affirmation and admiration, creating a cycle of dependency on external validation. This behavior can manifest through excessive sharing of personal milestones or achievements, often overshadowing the contributions or experiences of others. For those trying to identify narcissism in their social circles, paying attention to how individuals interact with their online audience can provide insights into their true nature.

Moreover, the anonymity and distance afforded by online interactions can lead to more overt displays of narcissism. Individuals may feel emboldened to express their beliefs and opinions without the immediate social repercussions they might encounter in person. This can result in confrontational or dismissive behavior towards others, particularly in discussions where their self-image is challenged. Recognizing these patterns can help individuals identify potential narcissistic traits in acquaintances and even in closer relationships, as the online persona often reflects deeper psychological issues.

In professional settings, narcissistic traits can be particularly detrimental. Colleagues with narcissistic tendencies may dominate conversations, take credit for others' work, or manipulate group dynamics to maintain control. Their online behavior might include a focus on personal branding or an excessive emphasis on their professional accomplishments. Observing how individuals present themselves in professional online forums or networks can be telling. A consistent pattern of self-aggrandizing posts, coupled with a lack of recognition for team efforts, can indicate a narcissistic personality.

Finally, understanding the nuances of narcissism in the context of online behavior is crucial for those navigating relationships with narcissists. Strategies for coping may involve setting boundaries regarding online interactions and being mindful of the emotional impact of engaging with narcissistic individuals. By recognizing the signs of narcissistic behavior in digital spaces, individuals can better protect their mental health and establish healthier dynamics, both online and offline. This awareness can be particularly beneficial for individuals who find themselves repeatedly drawn into relationships marked by manipulation and self-serving behaviors.

The Influence of Social Media on Self-Perception

The influence of social media on self-perception has become increasingly significant in today's society, particularly among those navigating relationships with narcissists. Social media platforms serve as a double-edged sword, providing opportunities for connection while simultaneously amplifying feelings of inadequacy and comparison. Users often curate their online personas to present an idealized version of themselves, which can lead to distorted self-perceptions. For individuals dealing with narcissists, this curated reality can exacerbate feelings of self-doubt, as narcissists may leverage social media to showcase their own superior lifestyles, further manipulating those around them.

Narcissistic individuals are adept at using social media to reinforce their self-image. By selectively sharing achievements, attractive visuals, and glamorous experiences, they create a façade that can mislead others into viewing them as more successful or desirable than they truly are. This behavior can leave those in their orbit feeling inferior, as they compare their everyday realities to the polished versions presented online. The pressure to maintain a similar level of engagement can lead to an unhealthy cycle of validation seeking, where individuals may sacrifice their authenticity to gain approval from others, particularly from narcissists who thrive on admiration.

Moreover, the interactions that occur on social media can further entrench narcissistic behavior. Narcissists often use platforms to monitor the reactions of their followers, using likes and comments as a metric of self-worth. This dynamic can create a toxic feedback loop, where the need for external validation becomes paramount. Those dealing with narcissists may find themselves caught in this web, feeling compelled to engage in the same performance to garner recognition. This can lead to a distorted sense of self, where personal value is measured by online metrics rather than genuine self-acceptance.

The impact of social media on mental health is particularly concerning in relationships with narcissists. Increased exposure to unrealistic standards can contribute to anxiety, depression, and a diminished sense of self-worth. Those who are manipulated by narcissists may experience heightened emotional distress as they struggle to reconcile their authentic selves with the idealized images they encounter online. The constant comparison can erode self-esteem, making it increasingly difficult to escape the grasp of narcissistic influence and recognize one's inherent worth.

In conclusion, social media plays a pivotal role in shaping self-perception, especially for individuals entangled with narcissists. The curated nature of online interactions can distort reality and contribute to feelings of inadequacy, while narcissists exploit these platforms to reinforce their self-aggrandizing narratives. Recognizing the influence of social media is essential for those seeking to break free from narcissistic manipulation and reclaim their authentic selves. Navigating this landscape requires awareness, resilience, and a commitment to fostering genuine connections that honor one's true identity, rather than the superficial standards often perpetuated online.

8

Detecting Narcissism in Professional Settings

Interviewing and Hiring Red Flags

Interviewing and hiring individuals can be particularly challenging when dealing with narcissists. Recognizing red flags during the hiring process is essential for avoiding the pitfalls that can arise from bringing a narcissist into your professional environment. One major indicator is an applicant's tendency to dominate conversations. If the candidate consistently redirects discussions back to themselves, dismisses others' contributions, or engages in self-aggrandizing behavior, these traits can signal a narcissistic personality. It is crucial to note that while confidence is valuable, it should not overshadow the importance of collaboration and respect for others' perspectives.

Another red flag to watch for is the lack of accountability. Narcissistic individuals often deflect blame onto others, failing to take responsibility for their actions. During interviews, ask candidates about challenges they have faced and how they managed them. Pay attention to whether they acknowledge their role in any difficulties or if they shift the focus onto external factors. A candidate who cannot own their mistakes may cause significant disruption in team dynamics and can lead to a toxic work environment.

Inconsistency in behavior and responses can also indicate a narcissistic tendency. If a candidate presents themselves as exceptionally charming and agreeable during the interview but later reveals a pattern of hostility or defensiveness in follow-up interactions, this inconsistency may point to deeper issues. Narcissists are often skilled at putting on a façade to win over others, but their true nature may emerge once they feel secure in their position. It is essential to probe deeper and gather insights from multiple interviewers to identify any discrepancies in the candidate's presentation.

The use of language can be a significant indicator of narcissistic traits. Pay attention to the pronouns used by candidates; excessive use of "I" and "me" can indicate a self-centered perspective. Additionally, if they frequently describe past achievements in grandiose terms without acknowledging the contributions of others, this can reveal an inflated sense of self-worth. Effective team members should demonstrate a balance of self-promotion and humility, recognizing that collective effort often leads to success.

Finally, be cautious of candidates who exhibit a lack of empathy during the interview process. Empathy is a critical quality for collaboration and conflict resolution in any workplace. If a candidate struggles to understand or value the experiences of others, or if they express indifference towards the feelings of colleagues or clients, these traits can foreshadow future challenges in interpersonal relationships. By being vigilant about these red flags, organizations can better protect themselves from the negative impacts of hiring individuals with narcissistic tendencies, ultimately fostering a healthier work environment.

Team Dynamics and Narcissistic Influence

Team dynamics can be significantly affected by the presence of a narcissistic individual, whether in a workplace, social group, or familial setting. Narcissists often exhibit behaviors that disrupt collaboration and mutual respect, leading to an environment that prioritizes their needs over the collective goals of the team. This can manifest in various ways, such as undermining others, taking credit for achievements, or diverting attention to themselves during discussions. Understanding these dynamics is crucial for recognizing the influence of narcissistic behavior within a group context.

One of the key traits of narcissists is their ability to charm and manipulate those around them initially. They often present themselves as charismatic leaders, drawing people in with their confidence and assertiveness. However, this facade can quickly crumble as their self-serving behaviors become evident. Team members may find themselves feeling undervalued or exploited as the narcissist seeks to maintain control and power within the group. Identifying these behaviors early can help others set boundaries and protect their emotional well-being.

Moreover, the impact of narcissism on group dynamics extends to decision-making processes. Narcissists tend to dominate discussions and may dismiss the contributions of others, believing their ideas to be superior. This can lead to a toxic environment where team members feel hesitant to voice their opinions or contribute creatively. As a result, the team's overall effectiveness may decline, as collaboration and collective problem-solving are stifled. Recognizing these patterns is essential for fostering a healthier team dynamic where every member feels empowered to engage.

In romantic relationships, narcissistic influence can create an imbalance that affects both partners. The narcissist's need for admiration and validation can overshadow their partner's needs, leading to feelings of neglect and frustration. This dynamic can escalate into emotional manipulation, where the narcissist employs tactics such as gaslighting to maintain control. Understanding the signs of narcissistic behavior in intimate settings can help individuals navigate these challenges and seek healthier relationship patterns.

Finally, the role of social media in revealing narcissistic behavior cannot be overlooked. Narcissists often curate their online personas to emphasize their achievements and desirability, further perpetuating their need for validation and admiration. This can distort the perception of what constitutes a healthy relationship, as social media becomes a platform for comparison and competition. Recognizing the signs of narcissism in both online and offline interactions is vital for maintaining healthy boundaries and relationships, ultimately fostering a supportive environment free from manipulative influences.

Addressing Narcissism in Professional Development

Addressing narcissism in professional development is crucial for fostering a healthy work environment and promoting individual growth. Narcissistic behaviors can disrupt team dynamics, hinder collaboration, and create toxic atmospheres, making it essential to identify and address these traits early on. Understanding how to spot narcissistic tendencies among colleagues can empower individuals to take proactive measures to protect their professional development and mental well-being. By equipping oneself with the knowledge of what constitutes narcissistic behavior, employees can better navigate their interactions and mitigate potential conflicts.

In professional settings, narcissists often display certain traits such as a need for excessive admiration, a lack of empathy, and a tendency to exploit others for personal gain. These behaviors can manifest in various ways, including undermining colleagues, seeking credit for others' work, and dominating conversations. Recognizing these signs is the first step in addressing narcissism within the workplace. Training sessions and workshops that focus on identifying these traits can be instrumental in creating awareness among employees, allowing them to understand the dynamics at play and to develop strategies to cope with challenging situations.

Furthermore, it is essential to foster a culture of open communication and feedback within organizations. Encouraging employees to share their experiences and observations regarding narcissistic behavior can help create a supportive environment where individuals feel safe to discuss their concerns. Implementing regular check-ins and feedback mechanisms can provide valuable insights into team dynamics and highlight any problematic behaviors. Leaders should be trained to recognize and address narcissistic tendencies, ensuring that they are equipped to manage their teams effectively while promoting a culture of accountability and respect.

Professional development programs should also incorporate training on emotional intelligence and empathy. By enhancing these skills, employees can better manage their interactions with narcissistic individuals and reduce the negative impact of such behaviors on their mental health. Developing empathy can help in understanding the underlying motivations of narcissistic behavior, which can lead to more constructive responses rather than reactive ones. This shift can create a healthier work environment where individuals feel valued and respected, ultimately benefiting the organization as a whole.

Lastly, organizations must prioritize mental health and well-being in their professional development initiatives. The impact of narcissism on employees' mental health can be profound, leading to stress, anxiety, and decreased job satisfaction. By providing resources such as counseling services, stress management workshops, and opportunities for personal growth, organizations can help employees navigate the challenges posed by narcissistic behavior. A commitment to mental health not only supports those dealing with narcissists but also fosters a more resilient workforce that can thrive in the face of adversity.

9

The Impact of Narcissism on Mental Health

Effects on Victims of Narcissistic Abuse

The effects of narcissistic abuse on victims are profound and often long-lasting, permeating various aspects of their lives. Victims frequently experience emotional and psychological turmoil, which can manifest as anxiety, depression, and a diminished sense of self-worth. The manipulation and control exerted by narcissists create an environment where victims may question their perceptions and reality, leading to confusion and self-doubt. This psychological warfare can erode the victim's confidence, making it difficult for them to trust their instincts or make decisions without second-guessing themselves.

In romantic relationships, the effects of narcissistic abuse can be particularly devastating. Victims often find themselves trapped in a cycle of idealization and devaluation, where they are initially showered with affection and attention, only to be met with criticism and emotional neglect. This rollercoaster of emotions can lead to attachment issues and a fear of abandonment, as victims may become conditioned to believe they are unworthy of love and respect. The impact extends beyond the relationship itself, influencing future partnerships and hindering the victim's ability to form healthy, trusting connections.

In the workplace, victims of narcissistic abuse may endure a toxic environment that undermines their professional growth and mental health. Narcissistic leaders or colleagues often employ tactics such as gaslighting and favoritism, creating a culture of fear and competition. Victims may feel isolated and unsupported, leading to increased stress and burnout. The long-term implications can include decreased job satisfaction, productivity, and, in severe cases, career stagnation as victims grapple with the damaging effects of their experiences.

Among friends and family, the repercussions of narcissistic abuse can lead to strained relationships and a sense of betrayal. Victims may feel compelled to distance themselves from those who enable or exhibit narcissistic behaviors, leading to social isolation. The emotional toll can result in a pervasive feeling of loneliness and the belief that genuine connections are unattainable. Victims might also struggle with reconciling their love for the narcissist with the pain inflicted upon them, complicating their emotional landscape and further exacerbating feelings of confusion and despair.

Understanding the effects of narcissistic abuse is crucial for those navigating relationships with narcissists. Victims must recognize that their reactions and feelings are valid and that healing is a process that requires time and self-compassion. By acknowledging the profound impact of narcissistic behavior, individuals can begin to reclaim their sense of self and seek support from trusted friends or professionals. This journey toward recovery is essential not only for personal well-being but also for fostering healthier relationships in the future.

Coping Mechanisms and Support Systems

Coping with the challenges posed by narcissistic individuals requires effective mechanisms and robust support systems. For those navigating relationships with narcissists, whether in personal or professional spheres, understanding how to manage these interactions is crucial for maintaining mental health and personal well-being. It is essential to recognize that while narcissistic behavior can be manipulative and damaging, there are strategies that can help mitigate its impact. Establishing boundaries, practicing self-care, and seeking support from trusted individuals are foundational elements of coping effectively.

One of the primary coping mechanisms when dealing with narcissists is the establishment of clear boundaries. This involves defining what behaviors are acceptable and which are not, and communicating these limitations assertively. Narcissists often test boundaries, attempting to manipulate or control situations to their advantage. By being firm and consistent in enforcing boundaries, individuals can protect their emotional space and reduce the likelihood of being drawn into the narcissist's games. This practice of boundary-setting not only helps in personal relationships but is equally important in professional settings, where narcissistic behavior can disrupt team dynamics and undermine morale.

Self-care is another vital aspect of coping with narcissistic behavior. Engaging in activities that promote mental and physical well-being can serve as a buffer against the emotional toll of interacting with narcissists. This may include regular exercise, mindfulness practices, or pursuing hobbies that bring joy and fulfillment. Additionally, maintaining a healthy social life outside of the narcissistic relationship can provide necessary support and perspective. It is crucial to prioritize self-care as a means to counterbalance the negative effects of narcissism, allowing individuals to recharge and regain their sense of self.

Support systems play a pivotal role in coping with the complexities of narcissistic relationships. Connecting with friends, family, or support groups who understand the nuances of dealing with narcissists can foster a sense of validation and empowerment. Sharing experiences with others who have faced similar challenges can provide insights and strategies for navigating difficult interactions. Professional support, such as therapy, can also be instrumental in processing emotions and developing coping strategies tailored to individual circumstances. A therapist familiar with narcissistic dynamics can guide individuals in understanding their experiences and building resilience.

Lastly, recognizing the importance of education about narcissism can enhance coping strategies. Understanding the traits and behaviors associated with narcissism—such as manipulation, lack of empathy, and grandiosity—equips individuals with the knowledge to identify and address these behaviors more effectively. This awareness fosters a sense of control and agency in interactions with narcissists. By combining boundary-setting, self-care, support systems, and education, individuals can develop a comprehensive toolkit for managing the challenges posed by narcissistic relationships, ultimately leading to healthier dynamics and improved mental well-being.

Long-term Mental Health Consequences

Long-term exposure to narcissistic individuals can lead to significant mental health consequences for those who are targeted by their manipulative behavior. Victims may experience chronic stress, anxiety, and depression, which can stem from the constant emotional turmoil and invalidation inflicted by narcissists. The relentless need to appease or placate a narcissist can create a sense of perpetual unease, leaving individuals feeling trapped and powerless. Over time, this ongoing strain can manifest in physical symptoms such as fatigue, headaches, and sleep disturbances, further compounding the psychological impact.

One of the most pervasive effects of dealing with narcissists is the erosion of self-esteem. Narcissists often engage in belittling or gaslighting tactics, which can leave victims questioning their worth and abilities. This undermining of self-confidence can be profound and long-lasting, as individuals begin to internalize the negative messages they receive. The struggle to regain a sense of self can be a challenging journey, often requiring professional support and significant personal reflection to rebuild a healthy self-image.

Isolation is another critical consequence of narcissistic relationships. Narcissists frequently manipulate their victims into distancing themselves from supportive friends and family, fostering an environment of loneliness and despair. This isolation can exacerbate feelings of worthlessness and helplessness, making it even more difficult for individuals to seek help or find solace in external relationships. The lack of a support system leaves victims vulnerable, often leading to a downward spiral in their mental health.

In professional settings, the impact of narcissism can be equally detrimental. Victims may find themselves in a toxic work environment characterized by manipulation, favoritism, and a lack of recognition for their contributions. This can lead to burnout and disengagement, as employees struggle to navigate the complexities of working under a narcissistic leader or colleague. The cumulative effects of stress and frustration in the workplace can spill over into personal life, creating a cycle of discontent that permeates various aspects of an individual's existence.

Ultimately, recognizing the long-term mental health consequences of engaging with narcissists is crucial for recovery and healing. Awareness of these effects can empower individuals to seek appropriate support and develop strategies for disengagement. By understanding the manipulative tactics employed by narcissists, individuals can begin to reclaim their autonomy and rebuild their mental well-being, fostering resilience against the damaging influence of narcissism in their lives.

10

Tools and Techniques for Spotting Narcissism

Observational Techniques

Observational techniques are crucial for those dealing with narcissists, as they provide the tools necessary to identify manipulative behaviors and discern the true nature of individuals. One effective method involves careful attention to patterns of behavior rather than isolated incidents. Genuine narcissists often display consistent traits such as a lack of empathy, an exaggerated sense of self-importance, and a need for excessive admiration. By observing interactions over time, one can begin to see these patterns emerge, which can serve as a clear indicator of narcissistic tendencies.

In romantic relationships, the dynamics can be particularly complex due to the emotional investment involved. One should look for signs of manipulation, such as love bombing, where a partner may overwhelm with affection and attention initially, only to later withdraw affection or become critical. This cycle can create confusion and dependency, making it essential to observe how a partner responds to both positive and negative situations. Noting the balance of give-and-take in the relationship can help illuminate whether the individual exhibits narcissistic traits or is genuinely invested in the partnership.

In the workplace, narcissism can manifest in various ways, including the tendency to dominate conversations, dismiss the contributions of others, or take credit for collective successes. Observing interactions during meetings or collaborative projects can reveal who prioritizes their own interests over those of the team. Additionally, pay attention to how colleagues react to feedback and criticism; narcissists often respond with defensiveness or aggression, avoiding accountability for their actions. Recognizing these behaviors can assist individuals in navigating office dynamics and protecting their mental health.

When it comes to friends and family, the emotional ties can cloud judgment, making it vital to maintain a level of objectivity. Engage in reflective observation by noting how often interactions leave you feeling drained or inadequate. Genuine relationships should foster support and encouragement, whereas those with narcissists often involve manipulation and emotional turmoil. Keeping a journal of these interactions can provide clarity and help identify recurring themes of narcissistic behavior, enabling a better understanding of the relationship dynamics at play.

Lastly, the rise of social media has created a unique landscape for observing narcissistic behaviors. Online platforms often serve as a stage for overt displays of self-importance, including constant self-promotion and validation-seeking behaviors. Take note of how individuals curate their online personas and their reactions to social feedback. Understanding the role of social media in revealing narcissistic traits can provide valuable insights into a person's character. By employing these observational techniques, one can better navigate relationships affected by narcissism and protect their mental well-being.

Effective Communication Strategies

Effective communication is essential when dealing with narcissists, as it helps to establish boundaries, reduce conflict, and clarify intentions. Understanding the nuances of how narcissists communicate can empower individuals to navigate these challenging interactions more effectively. One fundamental strategy is to maintain a calm and assertive demeanor. Narcissists often thrive on emotional reactions; therefore, responding with composure can prevent them from manipulating the situation to their advantage. A steady tone and clear messaging can also reinforce your position, making it harder for them to divert the conversation or shift blame.

Another critical aspect of effective communication is active listening. While narcissists typically focus on themselves, demonstrating that you are genuinely engaged can create an opportunity for dialogue. This involves acknowledging their feelings or perspectives without necessarily endorsing their behavior. By validating their emotions without conceding ground, you can maintain your stance while reducing the likelihood of escalation. This approach can also help identify genuine narcissistic traits, as narcissists may struggle with empathy, often revealing more about themselves in the process.

Setting clear boundaries is paramount when communicating with narcissists. This means explicitly stating what behaviors are unacceptable and what the consequences will be if those boundaries are crossed. For instance, if a narcissistic colleague frequently interrupts you in meetings, addressing this directly and establishing a rule for respectful dialogue can help reduce such occurrences. Boundaries provide a framework for interactions and can deter narcissistic tendencies, as they thrive in environments where their behavior goes unchecked.

Moreover, it is crucial to be prepared for manipulation and gaslighting. Narcissists often employ tactics that distort reality, making it vital to stick to factual information and avoid getting drawn into emotional debates. Documenting conversations and maintaining a record of interactions can be beneficial, especially in professional settings where accountability is necessary. When faced with gaslighting, calmly reiterating the facts can help ground the conversation and remind you of your truth, rather than allowing the narcissist to create confusion.

Lastly, leveraging the power of support networks can significantly enhance communication strategies. Engaging with others who understand the dynamics of narcissism can provide valuable insights and emotional reinforcement. Whether through therapy, support groups, or trusted friends, sharing experiences can illuminate patterns and foster resilience. By recognizing that you are not alone in these encounters, you can approach communication with a sense of empowerment, ultimately leading to healthier interactions and improved mental well-being.

Resources for Further Learning

In navigating the complex landscape of narcissistic behavior, a variety of resources can provide invaluable insights and guidance. Books written by experts in psychology and interpersonal relationships often serve as foundational texts for understanding narcissism. Titles such as "Disarming the Narcissist" by Wendy T. Behary and "The Narcissist You Know" by Joseph Burgo offer practical strategies for recognizing and dealing with narcissistic individuals in various contexts, including friendships, family dynamics, and workplace interactions. These resources not only outline the characteristics of narcissism but also delve into the psychological underpinnings that inform such behavior.

Online courses and webinars are also excellent avenues for further learning. Platforms like Coursera and Udemy frequently offer courses focused on emotional intelligence, relationship dynamics, and personality disorders. Participating in these courses can enhance your ability to identify narcissistic traits and gain a deeper understanding of how they manifest across different types of relationships. Many courses feature interactive components, allowing participants to engage with instructors and peers, which can foster a supportive learning environment for those grappling with narcissism in their lives.

Support groups and forums, both online and in-person, can provide a communal space for individuals affected by narcissistic behavior. These platforms allow for the sharing of personal experiences and coping strategies, which can be incredibly validating and informative. Websites such as PsychCentral and the subreddit r/NarcissisticAbuse offer spaces where individuals can connect, share resources, and receive guidance from others who have faced similar challenges. Engaging in such communities can help individuals feel less isolated and more empowered to address the impact of narcissism in their relationships.

Professional therapy and counseling should not be overlooked as critical resources for those dealing with narcissists. Trained mental health professionals can offer tailored strategies to navigate the complexities of relationships with narcissistic individuals. Therapists can help clients develop personalized coping mechanisms, improve their communication skills, and enhance their emotional resilience. Additionally, they can provide a safe space for exploring the emotional toll that narcissistic relationships can take, facilitating healing and personal growth.

Finally, staying informed about the latest research in psychology can further equip individuals to recognize and combat narcissistic behavior. Academic journals, podcasts, and reputable mental health websites often publish articles and discussions that explore new findings in the field of narcissism. Following thought leaders and researchers on social media platforms can also provide ongoing education and updates about emerging trends in understanding narcissistic behavior. By actively seeking out diverse resources, individuals can build a comprehensive toolkit to help them identify and navigate the challenges posed by narcissism in various aspects of their lives.

11

The Influence of Narcissism on Group Dynamics

Narcissism in Group Settings

Narcissism in group settings can manifest in various ways, influencing dynamics and interactions among individuals. In any collective environment, whether in social circles, workplaces, or family gatherings, the presence of a narcissist can significantly alter the group's atmosphere.

Such individuals often seek attention and validation, which can lead to imbalances in power and communication. Recognizing these traits is crucial for those dealing with narcissists, as understanding their behavior can help mitigate the negative effects on group cohesion and morale.

One of the most observable traits of narcissists in group settings is their tendency to dominate conversations. They often redirect discussions to themselves, showcasing their achievements or experiences while disregarding the contributions of others. This behavior can lead to frustration among group members, who may feel undervalued or ignored. Spotting this pattern is essential, as it can reveal an individual's narcissistic tendencies, especially if they consistently seek the spotlight and show little interest in the input of others.

Narcissists may also engage in manipulative tactics to maintain control within a group. This can include gaslighting, where they distort facts or deny previous statements to confuse others and assert dominance. Such tactics can create a toxic environment, making it difficult for group members to express themselves or feel safe in their opinions. Recognizing these manipulative behaviors is vital for individuals who wish to protect themselves from the psychological toll that such interactions can impose.

In romantic relationships, the impact of narcissism can be particularly damaging. A narcissistic partner may use their charm initially to attract attention, only to later exhibit controlling or dismissive behaviors once the relationship is established. This dynamic can lead to emotional distress for the other partner, who may feel trapped in a cycle of validation-seeking and criticism. Understanding these patterns can empower individuals to identify red flags early on, fostering healthier relationship dynamics and personal boundaries.

The role of social media in revealing narcissistic behavior cannot be overlooked, as it provides a platform for individuals to showcase their lives and seek affirmation. Narcissists often curate their online personas to portray an idealized version of themselves, attracting followers and admiration. This can create a false sense of connection among group members, leading to envy or competition. Recognizing the influence of social media on narcissistic behavior can help individuals navigate their interactions more thoughtfully, fostering genuine relationships grounded in mutual respect rather than superficial validation.

Leadership and Narcissism

Leadership and narcissism often intertwine in complex ways, particularly in environments where authority and influence are paramount. Narcissistic leaders may initially appear charismatic and confident, drawing followers with their compelling vision and assertive demeanor. However, this facade often masks deeper insecurities and a relentless need for admiration. Understanding the juxtaposition of leadership and narcissism is crucial for those dealing with narcissists, as it helps to identify behaviors that can be detrimental to both personal well-being and organizational health.

In romantic relationships, recognizing narcissistic traits becomes essential for maintaining emotional balance. Partners of narcissists may find themselves in a cycle of idealization and devaluation, where their worth is contingent upon the narcissist's fluctuating need for validation. The narcissist's need for control can manifest in manipulative behaviors that undermine the partner's self-esteem. Understanding these dynamics can empower individuals to set healthy boundaries and seek support, ultimately leading to healthier relational choices.

Narcissism in the workplace can create toxic environments that hinder collaboration and productivity. Narcissistic leaders often prioritize their agendas over the team's needs, fostering a culture of fear and competition rather than support and innovation. This behavior not only stifles creativity but also contributes to high turnover rates and decreased morale. By recognizing the signs of narcissistic leadership, colleagues can better navigate these challenges and advocate for healthier workplace dynamics.

Among friends and family, the impact of narcissism can be particularly insidious. Narcissistic individuals may exploit familial bonds or friendships to maintain control and garner attention. This can lead to a cycle of emotional manipulation, where the narcissist's needs overshadow the well-being of others. Spotting these patterns early can help individuals protect their emotional health and maintain more balanced relationships, fostering an environment where mutual respect and support can thrive.

The role of social media in revealing narcissistic behavior cannot be overlooked. Platforms that allow for self-promotion can amplify narcissistic tendencies, as individuals curate their online personas to attract admiration. This behavior can distort perceptions of relationships and success, leading to unrealistic comparisons and feelings of inadequacy among peers. Understanding the influence of social media on narcissism is essential for developing a critical perspective on online interactions, enabling individuals to engage in healthier, more authentic connections both online and offline.

Group Decision-Making Challenges

Group decision-making can be particularly challenging in environments where narcissistic individuals are present. Narcissists often seek to dominate discussions, steering conversations in ways that elevate their status or validate their opinions. This behavior can create an imbalance in group dynamics, where the input of others is marginalized. As a result, group members may struggle to voice their perspectives or may feel pressured to conform to the dominant narrative set by the narcissist, leading to suboptimal outcomes for the collective decision-making process.

One significant challenge in group decision-making with narcissists is their tendency to prioritize personal gain over group objectives. This self-serving behavior can manifest as an unwillingness to compromise or collaborate, as narcissists often view themselves as superior to their peers. Consequently, they may manipulate discussions to ensure that their ideas are prioritized, disregarding the contributions of others. This undermines the collective intelligence of the group and can lead to resentment among members who feel undervalued or disrespected.

Another challenge arises from the narcissist's skill in deception and manipulation. They may employ tactics such as gaslighting or triangulation to create confusion and division among group members. This can lead to a breakdown in trust, making it difficult for the group to function cohesively. When decisions are influenced by fear or uncertainty, the quality of the outcomes is compromised. Members may become hesitant to share their thoughts, fearing backlash or ridicule, which further hinders effective decision-making.

Additionally, narcissists often thrive in competitive environments, which can exacerbate tensions within a group. Their need for admiration and validation can drive them to undermine others in pursuit of their own success. This competitive nature can create a toxic atmosphere where collaboration is stifled, and group members may feel pitted against one another. In such environments, the potential for innovative solutions diminishes, as individuals focus more on self-preservation than on working together towards a shared goal.

To navigate these challenges, it is essential for group members to recognize the signs of narcissistic behavior and establish strategies to mitigate its impact. Setting clear guidelines for discussions, promoting equal participation, and fostering a culture of respect can help counteract the negative influences of narcissists. Encouraging open communication and active listening can empower individuals to express their viewpoints, ultimately leading to more balanced and effective decision-making processes. By acknowledging the challenges posed by narcissism in group settings, individuals can better equip themselves to address these dynamics and foster healthier interactions.

12

Moving Forward

Setting Boundaries

Setting boundaries is a crucial step for anyone dealing with narcissistic individuals, whether they are friends, family members, or colleagues. Establishing clear and firm boundaries helps to protect your emotional well-being and prevents the manipulative behaviors typical of narcissists from infiltrating your life. The first step in setting boundaries is to identify what behaviors are unacceptable to you. This requires a deep understanding of your values and limits. By recognizing your triggers and knowing your non-negotiables, you can create a solid foundation for the boundaries you need to implement.

Once you have identified your limits, it is essential to communicate them clearly and assertively. Narcissists often thrive on ambiguity and may attempt to exploit any uncertainty you present. When you articulate your boundaries, do so using direct language and avoid apologizing for your needs. For example, if a friend frequently interrupts you or dismisses your opinions, you might say, "I need you to listen to me fully before responding." By asserting your boundaries, you are not only protecting yourself but also teaching the narcissist that their behavior will not be tolerated.

It is important to understand that narcissists may react negatively to your boundaries, often testing them to see how resolute you are. They may use guilt, manipulation, or even aggression to try to push you back into compliance. In these moments, it is vital to remain steadfast. Reaffirm your boundaries as needed and be prepared for potential backlash. This may involve emotional withdrawal or a temporary distancing from the relationship. Remember, your mental health and personal peace are paramount, and standing firm against a narcissist's attempts to breach your boundaries is essential for long-term well-being.

Setting boundaries is not a one-time event; it requires ongoing vigilance and adjustment. As your relationship with the narcissist evolves, so too may your boundaries. Regularly reassess your limits and be open to modifying them based on your experiences. If a boundary is consistently violated, it may be necessary to reconsider the relationship altogether. This process can be emotionally challenging, particularly if the narcissist is someone you care about deeply, but it is vital to prioritize your own needs and mental health.

Finally, it is beneficial to seek support while navigating the complexities of boundary-setting with narcissists. Connecting with others who understand the dynamics of narcissistic relationships can provide validation and encouragement. Whether through support groups, therapy, or trusted friends, having a network can bolster your resolve and offer practical strategies for maintaining your boundaries. Remember, setting boundaries is an act of self-respect and empowerment, equipping you to better manage the challenges presented by narcissistic individuals in your life.

Seeking Professional Help

Seeking professional help is an essential step for anyone dealing with narcissistic individuals, whether they are family members, romantic partners, friends, or colleagues. Recognizing the traits associated with narcissism can be the first step toward understanding the impact such relationships have on your mental health and well-being. However, understanding these traits is often not enough. Professional guidance can provide the support and strategies necessary to navigate these complex dynamics effectively. By seeking help from a qualified therapist or counselor, individuals can gain insights into their experiences and learn how to manage the emotional toll that narcissistic behavior can exert.

Therapists trained in dealing with narcissistic abuse can help clients identify the patterns of manipulation and control that narcissists often employ. This specialized knowledge is crucial as it empowers individuals to recognize when they are being gaslighted or emotionally manipulated. A mental health professional can facilitate discussions that clarify the difference between overt and covert narcissism, enabling clients to understand the subtleties of each and how they manifest in different relationships. This understanding is vital for individuals to regain a sense of agency and clarity in their interactions.

In romantic relationships, the emotional turmoil created by a narcissistic partner can be particularly debilitating. Professionals can provide tailored strategies for managing the emotional fallout from these relationships, equipping clients to set boundaries and prioritize their own mental health. Support groups, often facilitated by trained professionals, can also offer shared experiences that reassure individuals they are not alone in their struggles. These environments can foster healing and resilience, promoting a sense of solidarity among those who have endured similar challenges.

In workplace settings, the influence of narcissism can disrupt team dynamics and create toxic environments. Engaging with a psychologist or counselor can help professionals develop coping mechanisms to address the stress and anxiety stemming from such interactions. Understanding the traits of narcissistic behavior within a professional context can also lead to more strategic responses, reducing personal exposure to manipulation and allowing individuals to focus on their work without the burden of emotional distress. Additionally, workplace training programs led by professionals can educate employees on recognizing narcissistic traits, fostering a more supportive and aware organizational culture.

The role of social media in revealing narcissistic behavior cannot be underestimated, as online interactions often magnify these traits. Professionals can assist individuals in understanding how social media influences their perceptions of self-worth and relationships. By providing tools to critically analyze online interactions and the portrayal of others, therapists can help clients cultivate a healthier relationship with social media. In seeking professional help, individuals not only address the immediate challenges posed by narcissistic relationships but also embark on a journey toward greater self-awareness, empowerment, and healing.

Building a Support Network

Building a support network is crucial for anyone dealing with narcissistic individuals, whether in personal relationships, workplaces, or social circles. Establishing connections with people who understand the complexities of narcissism can provide a significant buffer against the emotional turmoil often inflicted by narcissistic behavior. A well-formed support network offers not only emotional validation but also practical advice and strategies for managing interactions with narcissists. It is essential to surround oneself with individuals who can offer perspective, encouragement, and a safe space to share experiences without judgment.

Identifying the right people to include in your support network is the first step. Look for friends, family members, or professionals who exhibit empathy and understanding of your situation. Those who can recognize and validate your feelings are invaluable, as they can help you differentiate between genuine concern and the manipulation often associated with narcissistic behavior. Seek out individuals who have experience dealing with narcissists themselves, as their insights can prove particularly beneficial. Establishing relationships with individuals who possess a clear understanding of narcissistic traits will help reinforce your perception of reality, which is frequently distorted by narcissistic manipulation.

It is equally important to maintain boundaries within your support network. While the goal is to receive support, it is essential to ensure that your network does not become a breeding ground for further dysfunction. Encourage open communication and foster an environment where everyone feels comfortable sharing their thoughts and feelings. This can help prevent any co-dependent relationships from forming, which can inadvertently mirror the dynamics experienced with narcissists. Establishing clear boundaries will also empower you to take ownership of your emotional well-being, preventing the unhealthy influences that can arise from interactions with narcissistic individuals.

In addition to personal connections, consider professional support as part of your network. Therapists, counselors, or support groups specializing in narcissistic abuse can provide critical tools and techniques for recognizing and coping with narcissism. These professionals can assist in developing strategies to navigate the complexities of relationships affected by narcissistic behavior, particularly in high-stress environments like workplaces. Engaging with others who have shared experiences can help reinforce feelings of solidarity and understanding, making it easier to confront the challenges posed by narcissists in various aspects of life.

Finally, leveraging technology and social media can enhance your support network. Online forums and groups dedicated to discussing narcissism can offer a wealth of knowledge and shared experiences. They provide a platform for connecting with others who have faced similar challenges, allowing for a broader exchange of strategies and coping mechanisms. However, it is vital to approach online interactions mindfully, ensuring that the spaces you engage with promote healthy discussions and do not contribute to further emotional distress. By building a robust and diverse support network, you can better equip yourself to handle the intricacies of dealing with narcissists and safeguard your mental health in the process.

www.ingramcontent.com/pod-product-compliance
Lightning Source LLC
Chambersburg PA
CBHW072053150726
47999CB00005B/1752